How Potassium and Sodium Create an Alkaline Body

"Create an alkaline body to eliminate disease and produce superior health"

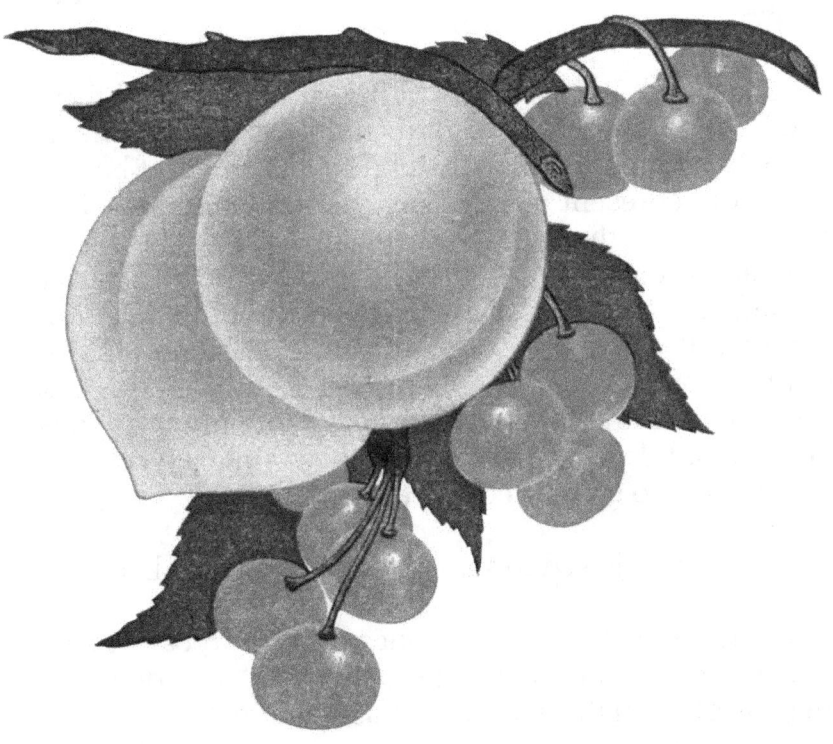

By Rudy S Silva, Natural Nutritionist

Table of Contents

Chapter 1: Introduction Potassium Health

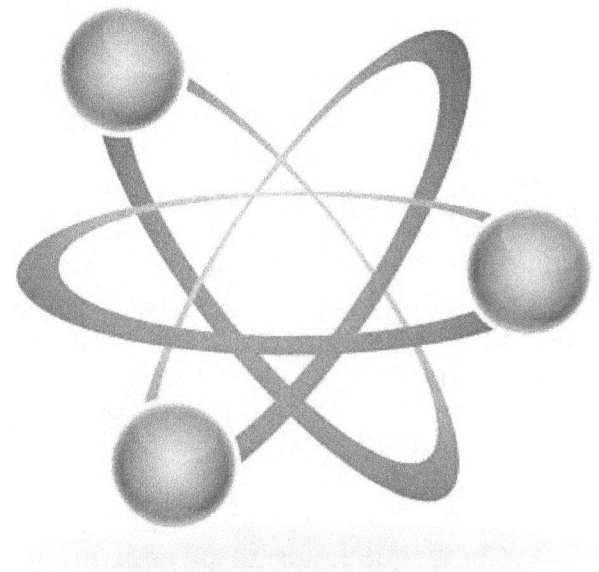

Get one of my best kindle books *free* by gong here:

http://natural-remedies-thatwork.com/optin.html

In this book, you will learn how and why potassium is used in your body. You will get a list of foods that you need to eat to get potassium and the type of potassium supplement you should take to keep healthy.

Potassium is another mineral that has many activities in your body, just like sodium. As potassium enters your body in food or by supplements, it is transformed into electrical charges called ions.

Potassium and sodium work together to maintain your body at a healthy level. One can't work properly without the other. But, potassium does other work that does not require the assistance of sodium. It helps other nutrients to help your muscles and nerves working like they should and to synthesize protein and store carbohydrates.

Potassium Ions

These potassium ions help create electrical potentials across cell membranes and along nerve path ways. What this potential, which is like a battery, does is create a condition where electricity flows where the potential is created carrying information and nutrients for your cells.

These nutrients that enter your cells come from the food you eat and are burned inside the cells with oxygen to create the energy you need to move around and for all your body functions.

Potassium is an element that is needed and found in all tissues and cells of your body. It helps to provide smooth function and activities for these cells. It is called an intercellular nutrient since is found mostly inside the cell liquid.

Potassium is found in all foods, but it's easier to absorb it from vegetables and fruits.

The Great Alkalizer

Potassium is also known as the "Great Alkalizer" since it easily combines with phosphorus, chlorine, and sulphur, which are all acid residue elements. If you have a slight potassium excess in your body, you will have stamina, good body movement, and may have excellent thought processes. Athletes are potassium people because of the precise body movements, speed and energy they use. Potassium gives them body and brain health.

It is known that plants need potassium in the soil to grow healthy. Potassium protects plants from diseases and germs, and it does the same thing in your body. It helps to make your body alkaline and brings in more oxygen into your cells for more protection against germs that like a low oxygen environment. It keeps your blood at a high alkaline level.

Potassium Losses

Your body needs all the potassium you can eat, and on occasion you will need to take a supplement. Any excess potassium that you have will be excreted in your urine. Your kidneys determine how much potassium should be in your body. If your kidneys are weak or diseased, it may excrete too much potassium through your urine, or it may maintain too much in your body.

Severe loss of potassium can initiate a heart attack. However, very few people ever reach this condition.

If your body retains too much potassium, then this upsets the balance of minerals in your body. One result is less calcium will be absorbed and used by your body.

If you do any type of athletic training or physical activity, such as running, bike riding, tennis, and other activities, feeling dizzy or faint during your activity can be related to a loss of potassium. This can be avoided by eating foods that give you a good balance of minerals and perhaps having an electrolyte drink before you practice that does not have sugar.

You can lose potassium when you vomit, have diarrhea, use laxatives or diuretics, sweat excessively, or have surgical drainage.

You can also lose or excrete potassium, if you take drugs. Here is a list of drugs that cause you do lose potassium.

Amphotericin, Antifungals
Antiparkisonism Medicines
Aspirin
Bronchodilators
Corticosteroids, Prednisone, Prednisoione
Digitalis
Diuretics
Penicillin
Tetracyclines
Ulcer medications
Sedatives
Antacids
Anticonvulsants
Stool softeners
Cough Cold Remedies

Potassium and Disease

Potassium is the main ion that is inside your cells, and sodium is the main ion outside your cells. This is what makes the electrical potential across your cell membrane causing nutrients to move into the cell and toxin to move out.

If you lack potassium, you can easily build it back up with food or supplements. When your body stores of potassium get too low, and it is expressed as low blood potassium, this can be a life threatening condition.

It is believed by herbalists that people with cysts, tumors, moles, and warts have a deficiency of potassium.

It was discovered by Dr. Gerson, The Gerson Therapy, that all people that have a chronic disease are low in potassium.

When an excess of Na+ is in your cells where potassium should dominate, production of body enzymes is decreased. This condition also disturbs the electric potential across the cells leading to malfunction of cellular activities.

To counteract the lack of potassium drinking plenty of fresh vegetable and fruit juices is what is required. This can also be done with a good source of potassium supplements, but drinking juices provides you with more minerals that you might be lacking.

Chapter 2: Potassium and Sodium In Your Body

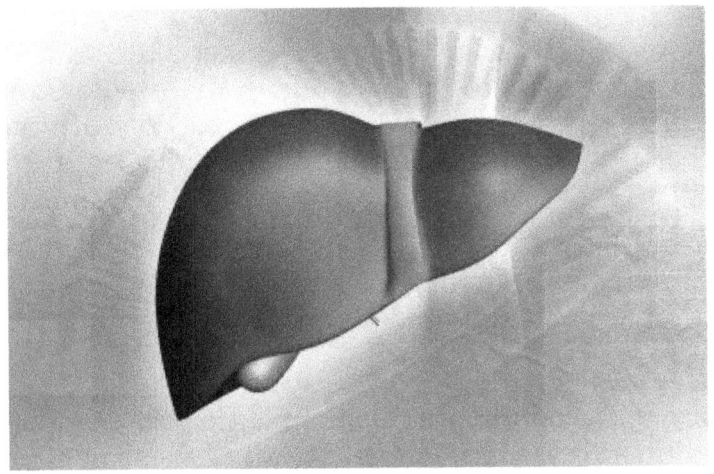

Potassium has a strong influence in the function of the liver and is regulated in your body by iodine. The real function of iodine is to move potassium, and the iodine may have to come from only organic iodine found in natural food to do this.

Since potassium is regulated in the liver, this happens around 2 am in the morning. If you wake up at 2 am in the morning, it's an indication that you have an imbalance in potassium. This imbalance most likely will be the use of some medication. Waking up at 3am in the morning indicates a calcium or magnesium deficiency.

The ratio of potassium to sodium in your body is the critical part that has to be maintained so that you have maximum health. Raw foods such as fruits and vegetables have the natural potassium to sodium ratio that needs to be maintained. When you cook this produce, you destroy this ratio and your body finds it hard to recognize this food as good for your body. This affects your well-being and future health.

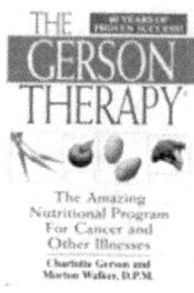

In The Gerson Therapy, 2001, New York, Charlotte Gerson and Morton Walker, D.P.M., point out, "In his monthly newsletter Health & Healing, Julian Whitaker, M.D. writes, 'The way to bring your sodium-potassium ratio back into balance is to eat lots of vegetables, legumes, whole grains, and fruits. These wholesome foods naturally have an excellent sodium-to-potassium ratio of a least 1:50.' Dr. Whitaker adds that some fruits, such as oranges, offer a good mineral proportion of 1 part sodium to 260 parts potassium."

Potassium and sodium are the main ionic minerals that create the Sodium Potassium Pump in your cell structure, which allows cells to receive nutrients for cell function and to eliminate toxins and other nutrients from within the cells.

Potassium easily dissolves in water. When it does, it becomes ionized and is an electrically charged molecule. It has one loose electron in its outer orbit and this electron can easily move on to another element or molecule. When this happens, it creates and electrical current. In this ionic form, potassium is call and electrolyte.

Potassium in your body

There is only 3-4 oz. of potassium in your body at one time. But this small amount creates a body that can recover from disease or injuries quickly. It does this by using albumin, casein and fibrin to repair and rebuild areas and to bring in more oxygen to the injured area.

Your body increases in efficiency when you have the excess

potassium. Here are some of the benefits of potassium:

Enzyme production
Improves elimination of wastes
Increases arterial and venous circulation
Improves sexual function
Improves heart function
Improves nervous system and brain performance
Controls cell life and function
Alkalizes the blood and the body
Maintains nerve electrical conduction
Improves hair growth
active in skin health
Promotes fibrin
Controls muscle coordination
Reduces internal oxidation
Reduces pain
Reduces intercellular edema
Improves vigor and reduces low energy levels
Reduces aches and pains
Reduces anxiety
Maintains heart beat

Improves Hair Growth

When you have a lot of potassium in your body, your chances of going bald are less. Your roots are stronger, and your hair stands are thicker. If you're a women, your hair will grow longer and stronger.

Controls muscle coordination

Strong, muscular, and athlete men have a lot of potassium in their body. The high level of potassium gives them a strong nervous system, good nerve function, and brain activity. This occurs because potassium attracts oxygen. This excess oxygen gives these people the energy to perform all their athletic activities.

Improves Elimination of Wastes

When you have excess potassium, the kidneys remove it from your blood. Potassium is also removed from your body through tears, perspiration, and fecal matter. Potassium is also used up in combining with phosphorous, chlorine, and sulfur.

When you lack potassium in the colon, the waste in the colon starts to ferment and putrefy, and this feeds the bad bacteria and allows them to multiply. With the addition of body heat, this fermenting matter produces gases, toxins and acids that get re-absorbed back into your bloodstream. The lack of potassium in your body will produce auto-intoxication and cause self-poisoning.

Cancer

In the case of cancer, it is important to keep high levels of potassium in the body with a reduced intake of table salt to prevent the formation of new tumors.

Fibrocystic Tumors

Fibrocystic tumors are made of potassium. When potassium is in balance in your body, your body will have normal function. Potassium has to be in balance with sodium, cesium, rubidium, iodine, and lithium.

Chapter 3: How Potassium Prevents Diseases

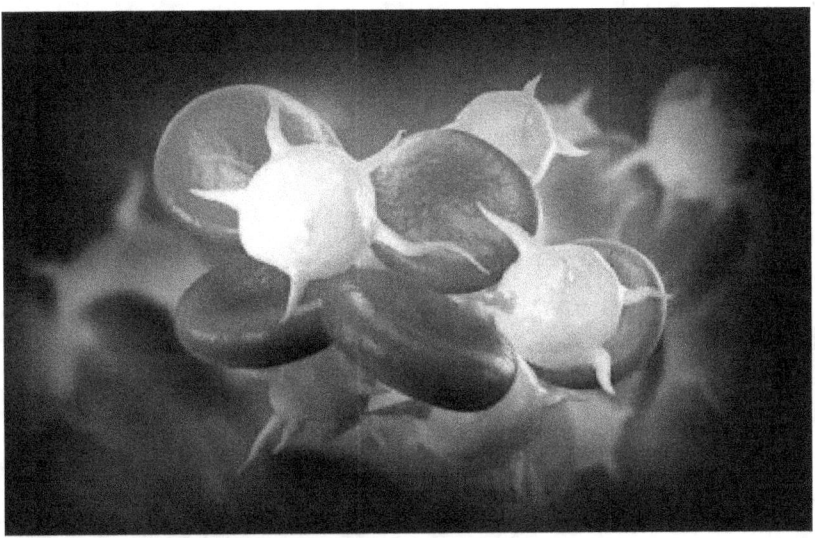

Alkalizes the blood and the body

Remember that the body's pH should be in the range of 7.4, which makes the body alkaline. Potassium is known for its ability to neutralize body acids and keep your body at 7.4 pH.
In addition, Potassium and sodium chloride work in all areas of your body to neutralize acids and toxins. Potassium chloride is mostly found in your muscle tissues, red blood cells and nerve tissues where it neutralizes acids created during physical activities.

When the pH in the liquid outside your cells drops, potassium inside the cells comes out to bring the liquid pH back up to normal.

Acid Binding

There are certain minerals that are called acid binding. And these minerals found in fruits and vegetables are sodium, potassium, chloride, calcium, phosphorus, magnesium.

What acid binding means is when you eat fruits with these minerals, they will seek out acids in your body and combine with them to neutralize them by creating a new chemical called alkaline forming ash.

Alkaline Ash

Now, this alkaline forming ash has tied up an acid and is carried to the kidney where it is expelled as urine. Of course, acids in the body are toxic, so the body has the priority of getting rid of them fast, since they can damage tissue and cause pain and disease.

So, you can see the importance of getting a lot of alkaline minerals into your body. Without them, acids which do not get bonded to an alkaline mineral would move into body tissue and continue their body damage. Having an excess of acid in your body results in what is called an acid body. An acid body occurs when you don't have enough fruits and vegetables in your diet.

It is believed that cancer lives and thrives better in an acid body, which means a body liquid of 7.0 pH or lower. And, when your blood pH leans towards an acid condition, your nervous system and brain start to slow down. Liquid is acidic when its pH is between 1.0 to 6.99 pH.

Potassium also works to:

Reduce stomach acids
Reduce intestinal acids
Improve stomach, intestinal, and colon peristalsis

Increases the alkalinity of cells, blood, lymph, body fluids and solids

Improves heart action
Improves Arterial pressure
Stabilizes blood pressure and circulation
Promotes good kidney action
Calms the heart and nerves
Prevents constipation and dehydration
Improves the activity of the adrenal and pituitary glands
Combines with albumin to form brain gray matter

Controls Muscle Coordination

When you use muscles as you do various activities, you produce monopotassium phosphate, lactic acid, and carbon dioxide. If you do not eliminate these acids, muscles will function properly. Potassium is necessary to eliminate these acids. Potassium salts such as potassium chloride and sodium chloride are necessary in your muscle's structure so that glycogen can be converted to muscle energy so that you can have good muscle movement and strengthen.

Reduces Pain

Potassium is a natural pain reducer which helps to control headaches, uterine pains, convulsions, and neuralgia. It helps to give you sound sleep and promote nerve action. It helps you to reduce anxiety, stress, worry, fear, and grief. All sorts of issues related to over excitement are reduced by potassium, such as excess sexual excitement, hysterical convulsions, or uterine convulsions.

Excesses of Potassium

When you have slight excess of potassium in your diet or in

your body, this is not a problem. It is quickly used up, since it works through your whole body to provide you with powerful muscle action, mental capability, calming action of the heart and mind, and powerful eyesight.

But, when you have too much potassium, it has a weaken effect in your body. It has a paralytic effect on your autonomic nervous system, the motor and sensory nerves and brain functions. An excess of potassium causes a reduction in sodium and chlorine by causing their precipitation.

Excess potassium will cause thought confusion and weak reasoning and unfounded ideas. Imagination and creativity are dulled, and memory becomes reduced. Excess blood moves to brain areas that cause wild and violent impulses.

You will see an increase in pulse rate, and blood pressure, when you have an excess potassium. In addition, you will have excess urination, perspiration, and muscle weakness.

Excess potassium attacks hemoglobin, causes vomiting, stomach pains, cramps, heart failure, coma, jaundice, convulsions, diarrhea, skin ulcers, tissue dryness, and skin pustules.

You can accumulate excess potassium when you eat preserved meats. Use drugs that contain potassium bromide, potassium phosphate, potassium carbonate, or potassium sulphate. If you eat a diet high in potassium or take an excess of potassium supplements you can also accumulate an excess of potassium in your body.

Having excess potassium in your body is not a common situation, since the kidneys will remove excess potassium and excrete it. But, when you have kidney malfunction, this can lead to excess potassium, if you are eating a diet high in potassium or are taking potassium supplements. A deficiency in potassium is more typical, since most people may not eat foods high in potassium or take potassium supplements. And, on occasion the kidney can excrete potassium even when you are low in body potassium.

Potassium deficiency

If you lack potassium in your body, you need to correct this condition right away. Blood tests and your doctor can help you determine if you have low blood potassium. Some of the symptoms of low level potassium are:

Appetite loss
Muscle cramps
A state of confusion
Mild to severe constipation
Excretion of calcium in urine

Improving Heart Function

If potassium deficiency is not taken care of, your heart will become irregular, causing a decrease in the blood being pumped into your body. This condition can lead to a stroke or heart attack.

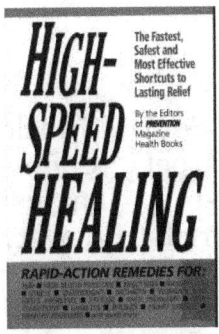

In their book, High Speed Healing, Editors of Prevention Magazine Health Books, 1991, Pennsylvania, reported that, "Potassium-rich foods have been shown to lower blood pressure, and a deficiency of potassium - whose chemical symbol is K – has been linked to an increase in blood pressure. Fresh fruits and vegetables – especially bananas and potatoes– dry beans, and whole grains are rich in potassium, says potassium expert George, Webb,

Ph.D., an associate professor of Physiology and biophysics at the University of Vermont Medical College.

In one study, 859 people over a 12-year period reduced their risk of dying from stroke by 40 percent by eating just one extra serving of fresh fruits or vegetables a day. And the more potassium – rich foods they ate, the lower their risk."

The reason high blood pressure is controlled by potassium is that it can restore normal kidney function.

The kidneys play an important function in blood pressure.

If you are on are on any type of diuretic medication, you will tend to lose potassium. If you have a severe case of diarrhea or a long-standing diarrhea, you will also be losing potassium that your body needs.

Potassium is one of the superstars for lowering high blood pressure and cholesterol.

In other studies, it was shown that some men, after a year on a high potassium diet, could reduce their high blood medication by 50%. And, other men, in the study, were able to stop their drug medication completely. This was done by having 3 to 6 servings of high-potassium foods every day.

Stroke

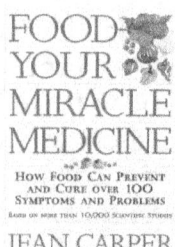

In her book called, Food Your Miracle Medicine, Jean Carpet, Harper Collins Publishers, 1993, reports on this study, "Eat just one extra serving of a potassium-rich food every day; that too may reduce your risk of stroke by 40 percent. That's what researchers discovered by analyzing the diets of a group of 859 men and women over age 50, living in southern California. The investigators documented that small differences of potassium in the diet predicted who would die of a stroke twelve years later.

Remarkably, nobody with the highest intake of potassium, more than 3,500 mg a day, died of a stroke. However, those who regularly ate the least potassium, less than 1950 mg, per day had much higher fatal stroke rates than all the others.

Among those who skimped the most on potassium, the odds of stroke deaths shot up 2.6 times in men and 4.8 times in women. Further, the more potassium-rich foods the subjects ate, the fewer strokes they had.

Indeed, the researchers concluded that with every extra daily 400 mg of potassium in the food, the odds of a fatal stroke dropped 40 percent."

Alcoholics

People who are alcoholics, have poor diets, are anorexic tend to be deficient in potassium. If you are on a diuretic drug, you will lose potassium and eating potassium foods will be of no value, since they will be excreted.

Respiratory Illness

When you have too much salt in your diet, you get your potassium sodium ratio out of balance. This will affect your nervous system. Since your nervous system controls your respiratory system, this can lead to a variety of respiratory illnesses such as emphysema or bronchitis.

Potassium obtained from vegetable soups, fruits, or supplements has a laxative effect in the colon.

Kidney Stones

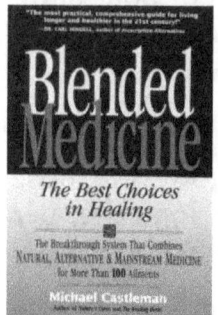

In Blended Medicine, Michael Castleman, Rodale, 2000, says that, "At the Kaiser Permanente Medical Care Program in Oakland, California, Brue, Ettinger, M.D., gave 64 people with recurrent kidney stones either a supplement containing potassium and magnesium citrate or a placebo. After 3 years, the supplement takers had 85 percent fewer recurrences than the placebo takers.

For her patients, clinical nutritionist Shari Lieberman Ph.D. prescribes 200 milligrams of potassium and 500 milligrams of magnesium every day. Because of potential serious risks associated with potassium, take supplements only under your doctor's care."

Muscle Cramping

When you exercise or do some activity that you typically don't do, your muscles can become sore or cramp. This can occur when you don't have enough minerals to neutralize the lactic acid that is created during your exercise.

When you develop this kind of soreness, you can take a supplement of potassium with calcium and magnesium. A better way to get the potassium you need is to eat potassium rich food and then add your calcium magnesium capsules.

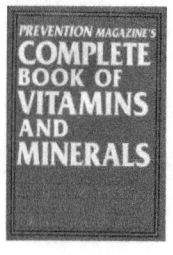

In Prevention Magazine's Complete Book Of Vitamins and Minerals, Rodale Press, 1988, they say that, "There is far from a consensus on the effects of mineral loss in exercise, but add a few more to the list of nutrients to monitor. Potassium, magnesium and zinc are lost in sweat, though losses vary widely from one person to the other. A nutrition expert and a runner himself, Gabe Mirkin, M.D., coauthor of the Sports Medicine Book, says exercisers who feel weak and tired may be suffering from 'the mineral blues,' a deficiency of potassium and magnesium inside muscle cells. When Dr. Mirkin, who ran 100 miles a month, suddenly found that running a quarter-mile 'felt like a marathon,' he had his blood tested. He learned that he was potassium deficient, something he remedied with copious quantities of fruit juices."

Diabetics

Potassium assists iodine in creating thyroid hormones, which increase the metabolism and regulate the metabolism of glucose.

Constipation

Because potassium is involved in muscle contractions and function, the lack of potassium can lead to constipation. The severity of the reduced peristaltic colon action will depend on the deficiency in potassium and the length of this deficiency.

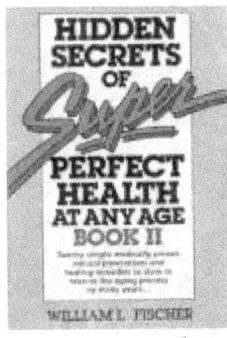

In Hidden Secrets of Super Perfect Health At Any Age Book II, William L. Fischer, Fischer Publishing Corporation, Ohio, 1986, writes, "Persons on a refined, denatured diet deficient in potassium quickly develop fatigue, listlessness, gas pains, constipation, insomnia and low blood sugar. Muscles become soft and flabby and the pulse becomes slow, week and irregular. By far, the greatest harm caused by a lack of potassium is the effect on the heart. Heart attacks are often associated with a low potassium intake.

An excessive intake of sodium, salt, can produce a potassium deficiency even when it appears the diet is adequately supplied. Yeast is an incomparable source of needed potassium. "

Chapter 4: Foods high in potassium

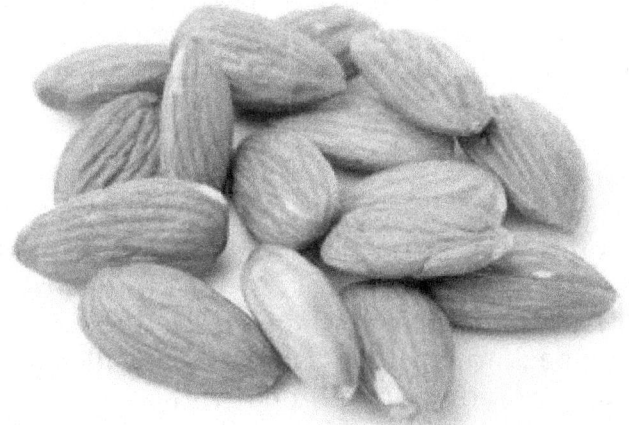

One reason you may be low in potassium is that when you boil vegetables, you lose the potassium into the water or it's lost with the steam. Of course, one way to minimize this loss is to drink the liquid you use in boiling.

Potassium Cocktail

This works out ok when you make a soup or when you create a potassium cocktail as outlined in Health Tonics, Elixirs and Potions, Carlson Wade, 1971, New York,

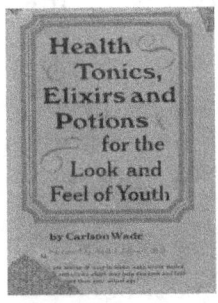

"Select sun dried fruits such as apricots, prunes, raisins, pears, and peaches. Be sure to obtain sun-dried fruits that have not been chemically dried or treated. These are available at health stores. Heat a kettle of water. After it bubbles, turn off heat and let the water simmer down. Next, place an assortment of sun- dried fruits in a deep bowl, cover, then simmer in water. Place a cover on the bowl. Let it remain at room temperature overnight. In the morning pour off one or two cups of the juice and drink. This is your Potassium Cocktail. You may eat the fruit for breakfast. This Potassium Cocktail has a power packed mineral benefit that is reportedly second to none for its effectiveness in rejuvenating the blood stream and recreating the sought-after look and feel of youth."

Potassium Broth

Here is another way to create a highly concentrated drink or liquid of potassium. These cocktails or broths are a fantastic way to get back into balance when you lack potassium and are trying to get back to normally from a major illness. They not only provide you with potassium but with an array of minerals that helps you clean out your intestinal tract and to rejuvenate your blood.

In her book, The Body-Smart System, Helene, Silver, Bantam Books, 1990, outline a broth that you can create to use as stock broth or as a full meal. To do this, you need to do the following:

Gather These Vegetables,

14, carrots with tops, 14 celery stalks with tops, 2 bunches of beet tops, 4 potatoes, 2 onions, 4 cloves of garlic, 3 summer squash, 3 zucchini, 2 handfuls of parsley.

Place all chopped vegetables in a pot and cover with clean water, place a cover over the pot, boil and simmer for 30 minutes. After, turn heat off and allow to stand for another 30 minutes.

Remove the green tops from the vegetables and get rid of

them. Put the remaining vegetables into a blender, but add a little of the clear broth, 1/4 cup, into the blender to puree them.

Now you can use the pureed vegetables as a meal and the clear broth as stock broth for other soups.

You can refrigerate the unused parts and hold for up to 4 days.

Foods High In Potassium

The foods highest in potassium are sun dried black olives, potato peel broth, dulse, kelp, bitter greens, Irish moss. Other foods high in potassium are:

Almonds	kale	leafy green lettuce
Anise seeds	lentil	lima beans
Apples	parsley	dried pears
Bananas	beans	beets
Black cherries	pecans	raisins
Broccoli	rice bran	carrots
Sesame seeds	cashews	cucumbers
Dates	turnips	fish
Grapes	watercress	wheat germ
Wheat bran	tomatoes	spinach
Berries	oranges	garlic
Blackstrap Molasses	natural honey	avocado
Sardines	apricots	winter squash
Cantaloupe	sweet potato	yeast

Bananas

In his book, Arthritis Rx, Vijay Vad, M.D., Gotham Books, 2006, talks about bananas,

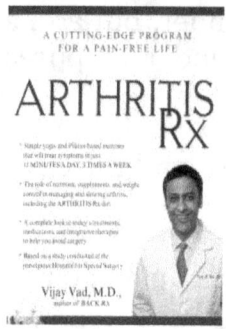

"Bananas are high in vitamin B6, potassium and iron. The FDA has endorsed the value of potassium: 'Diets containing foods that are good sources of potassium and low in sodium may reduce the risk of high blood pressure and stroke.' One study of 40,000 American male health professionals over four years determined that men who ate diets higher in potassium had a substantially reduced risk of stroke.

They [bananas] are also help with weight loss because they are rich in fiber, low in fat, and quite filling, and they feed the natural acidophilus bacteria in the intestines, necessary for proper digestion. What more could you ask from a delicious fruit that comes in its own wrapper?"

Yogurt

Plain yogurt is better nutritionally then milk. Eight ounces contain up to 40% of your daily calcium requirements. If you can't tolerate milk, you should be able to eat yogurt without any digestive problems.

Yogurt contains protein, calcium, potassium, phosphorus, vitamin B6, B12, niacin, and folic acid and is known to have just as much potassium as a banana.

Choose the yogurt that is labeled "sugar free, contains active, cultures, and/or plain yogurt." Remember that when yogurt is heat treated it loses most of it health benefits, since the heat kills the beneficial bacteria.

Potassium and sodium balance

When thinking about potassium, you need to think about

potassium and sodium balance. Potassium does not work independently in your body and must be brought into your body in food that is balanced with sodium. This balance is only found in raw, unpreserved fruits and vegetables. In your body, a specific ratio of potassium and sodium must be maintained so that you can have the best health.

Most produce has 20 times more potassium than sodium. In your body, it has 3 times more potassium than sodium.

Your body finds it easy to excrete potassium, since it comes out of your urine, sweat, fecal matter, tears, and in all other types of body secretions. However, your body tends to hold on to sodium, so if you have an excess of sodium this will affect your potassium-sodium balance.

Most fruits and vegetables are low in sodium and in a natural diet containing raw fruits and vegetables, the body would be low in sodium and that is why it holds on to sodium.

But, when eating processed foods, which are high in sodium, your body ends up having high sodium content, thereby changing the potassium – sodium ratio, which leads to disease.

Your kidney will excrete 10 mg of sodium, if you are low in sodium, but will excrete up to 240 mg of potassium, since normally, you have more potassium than sodium in your body.

You will notice that most processed food has high sodium content. Salt is used as a preservative and helps to inhibit molds and bacteria and to help food keep its color. The use of salt is saving manufacturer tremendous money while causing you untold bad health.

Eating these foods will create an imbalance your potassium to sodium ratio. Slight good changes in what you eat and the way you eat will improve your body's potassium – sodium balance. Here is a small list of foods that are out of balance and contain from 2 to 10 times more sodium than potassium, the reverse of what it should be:

Apple pie	white bread	cheese spreads
Cheese	cold cuts	cottage cheese
Dry cereal	frankfurters	green olives
Pancakes	peanut butter	canned peas
Potato chips	Ritz crackers	canned salmon
Saltines	sauerkraut	canned tuna

Reduce your salt intake by using herbs to season your food. Always look at the content of the food you buy. Buy more those foods that don't have added salt. Instead of salt on your eggs try using coriander, parsley, tarragon, thyme, or basil. Use herbs to season your chicken or fish.

Try to get more potassium into your diet than you do salt. Use raw fruits and vegetables. You can cook vegetables slightly and still maintain a good ratio. Eat raw nuts. Best nuts to eat are almonds, pecans, and pine.

Here is a list of good foods and the milligram amount of potassium they have in 100 gram.

Dulse	8060
Kelp	5273
Irish moss	2844
Pistachio nuts	972
Dehydrated prunes	940
Sunflower seeds	920
Dried lentils	790
Raisins	763

Parsley	694
Avocado	604
Yams	600
Spinach	470
Potato with skin	407
Banana	370
Carrots	340

Here is a list of foods or body conditions that will deplete your stored body potassium:

- Alcohol
- Antibiotics
- Diarrhea
- Caffeine
- Diuretics
- Sweating
- High cholesterol
- Cortisone
- Aldosterone
- Pain and inflammation products
- Laxatives
- Salt
- Stress
- Sugar

Chapter 5: Using potassium supplements

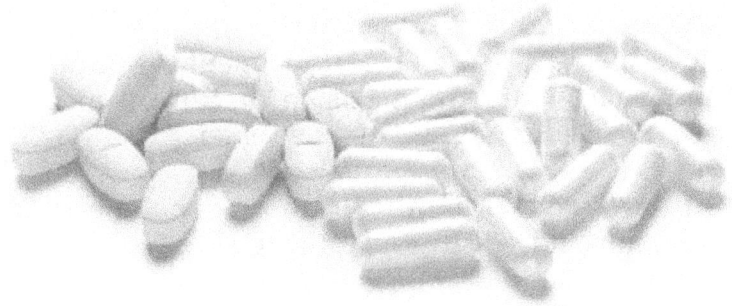

Potassium supplements may be prescribed by your doctor when you have chronic diarrhea, excess vomiting, high blood pressure, over use of laxatives, or diabetic acidosis.

Take caution when using potassium supplements, since there are dangers with overdosing. If you are on medication or are not in good health, then it is best to see a doctor before taking potassium supplements.

Use food first to get more potassium. Food is very high in potassium, and you can easily increase your intake of potassium to 5000mg by picking the right foods. Typically, you may want to increase your potassium to around 3000mg for general maintenance.

When using potassium supplements, always take them with meals. Potassium requires other minerals and vitamins to be present for adequate digestion and adsorption. The actual form you use is important so that your body will be able to absorb it.

If you feel you are low in potassium it is a good idea to ask your doctor for a nutritional blood test for potassium and other minerals. In this way, you know for sure if you are low and need to work on this part of health.

When you are on a diuretic, you deplete your potassium, so it's a good idea to add a potassium supplement to your diet. Take this supplement with your meals so that it can mix with the other vitamins and minerals you have eaten.

Potassium glycerophosphate – is one of the best forms of potassium, since it is easily and quickly absorbed by your body and cell walls.

Potassium citrate – is readily absorbed, and it is useful in restoring urinary citrate back to normal. Citrate is important because it reduces the formation of calcium salt stones. In the urine, citrate can be reduced when you eat excess sodium and protein. In addition, Potassium citrate reduces urinary calcium excretion, which helps lessen the loss of calcium.

Potassium aspartate – is a form where potassium is tied to the aspartic acid, which is an acidic amino acid. When minerals are tied to amino acids they pass easily and quickly through your intestinal wall and into your blood stream.

Potassium Chlorine - is a salt substitute and may be found in some supplements. It is not a good idea to use potassium chlorine in place of sodium chlorine, table salt, since after potassium is used up the chlorine can combine sodium and thereby reducing the sodium available to work with potassium in the Potassium Sodium Pump. Also, Potassium Chlorine interferes with the adsorption of vitamin B12.

When taking potassium supplements, make sure the formulation also has magnesium. Magnesium is necessary to maintain potassium in the body. Also, your heart muscle will not hold potassium without the presence of magnesium.

Final Comments

Potassium works with sodium to create the Potassium-Sodium Pump that allows nutrients to enter each cell. The Pump also allows toxic and other waste to exit the cell. When the body is low in calcium, calcium is pulled out of storage from the cell interior and out into the body where it is needed.

When you are deficient in potassium, you will experience body weakness and tiredness. Your mental abilities will diminish, and your nervous system will suffer from reduced nerve transmissions.

Building up excess potassium in the body has similar effects as not having enough. It is best to add those raw foods that have the proper potassium to sodium ratio, especially if you have a diet high in processed foods. Using potassium supplement must be done with caution. If you do use them, use low doses so you can see the results. You can take your saliva pH and then measure it again after a week of supplements to check your progress.

Things for you to do

Look at the list of foods high in potassium and add at least 3 to 4 of them to your daily or weekly diet. As usual, check your saliva pH and then do it again after a week of using more potassium foods.

To get more potassium in your diet you can take from 100mg to 500mg per day. The higher dose is for when you are dealing with high blood pressure or other illnesses. Just to increase your potassium intake, use 100 - 200mg per day.

Part 2: Sodium Nutrition Diet Revealed

"What You Need To Know About Sodium, So It Can Give You a Pain-Free Life"

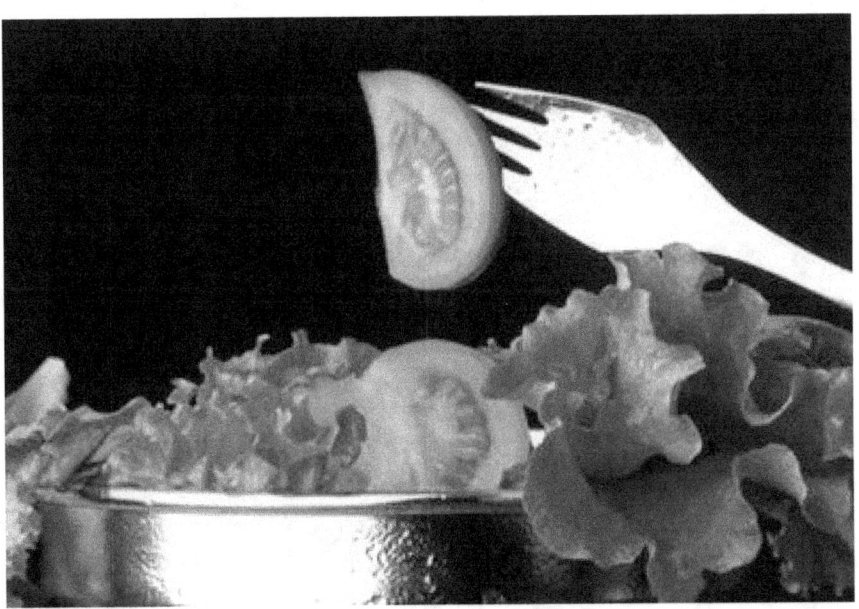

Chapter 6: Sodium The Youth Element

"Sodium is considered the Youth Element, since in the right proportions in your body, it will keep you young"

Your body has amazing ways that it can prolong your life. Many people and scientist look at the body from a chemical view point, but in fact, it is an electrical body.

In his book, The Philosopher's Stone, Michiio Kushi recounts how he performed an experiment in his laboratory where he transmuted sodium, Na+ into Potassium, K+. Having the right sodium in your body can provide transmutation when you need it.

In this book, you will discover why you should be concerned about sodium foods and your sodium diet and how this is related to potassium. In the end, it's all about how you can have the best health by minimizing any health problems that can arise from having an imbalance of sodium with respect with other minerals.

Sodium, chloride, and potassium, calcium, magnesium and phosphorus are a few of the critical electrolytes or ions in your body. Sodium is a positive charged electrolyte that resides mostly outside of your body cells.

Sodium stands number one in importance in your body. Ninety percent of the sodium ions, Na+, that exist in the fluids outside of your cells are sodium. It is sodium that attracts fluids and water into the outer cellular area and maintains the balance of these fluids throughout your body.

Sodium is an alkaline mineral that has a positive charge like potassium that neutralizes acids, whereas potassium helps to drain acids out of the body. The chemical symbol for sodium ions is Na+ and for potassium it is K+. This indicates that Na+ lacks an electron in its outer orbit and will readily accept an electron so that it can be balanced electrically.

Since Chloride has one extra electron in its outer electron orbit, it can contribute this electron to sodium. The result is that sodium and chloride have an affinity for each other, and that is why you see NaCl as a product better known as table salt. You have approximately 3 ounces of sodium in your body.

In the presence of water, NaCl will dissociate into the ions Na+ and Cl-. When you eat food that contains sodium, your stomach acid will break down your food and in the process release the sodium in the food to form Na+. It is in this form that your body uses Na+, and it is found through out your body eliminating acid. It also serves to create electrical potentials across cell membranes, similar to small little batteries, that help to move nutrients across cell walls.

Many diseases are caused because people lack organic sodium, not table salt, in their diet and are deficient in it in their body liquids. Sodium is called the Youth Element, because if you always have the right amount in your body, you will be limber, pliable, and active. All athletic activities and active hobbies require your body to have plenty of sodium.

Organic Sodium

The difference between organic sodium and inorganic sodium, table salt, is organic sodium is found only in fruits and vegetables. It is alive and has electric magnetic energy and frequencies that your body uses to energize itself. But, inorganic sodium found in table salt and in many other processed foods and is considered dead food. Table salt is not alive and is not the correct sodium that the body needs for good health, but your body will still use it as a substitute when you lack organic salt.

Inorganic Sodium

Salt, sodium chloride, is not a food and is considered inorganic sodium. All inorganic substances are harmful to your body. Salt is crystal found in natural deep in the earth. It's mined and brought up to the surface where it is sorted and purified into various sizes. When it is dissolved by forcing water deep into the earth, it is called Brine.

Salt is used in many industries. It is used in thousands of applications from meat packers, food to leather processors. It is used to manufacture glass, soap, and paper. It is used in water, to build roads, refine metals, and make ice cream. It is not a food, but it is used as a seasoning in many foods.

Sodium in Your Body

Like calcium and potassium, sodium has many functions throughout your body and is stored throughout your body, for emergencies. It keeps calcium and magnesium in solution and prevents them from precipitating. It is active in the blood, lymph, lymph nodes, stomach, colon, cells, tissues, and wherever acid is formed in your body.

Sodium maintains the proper extracellular fluid volume, liquid outside cells, since it attracts water. If you have edema, excess water in your body, or high blood pressure, you need to back off on eating salt. When you don't have enough salt, you will lack water in your body. This has a dramatic effect on your blood pressure, since it will cause low blood pressure.

Sodium with the help of potassium and chloride transmits impulses in nerve and muscle fibers. All along nerve fibers, sodium exists creating an electric voltage across the nerve membranes, so that nerve impulses can travel to the various locations in your body.

Sodium is lost from your body in hot humid weather and when you do hard physical work. Sauna baths, fevers, sweating, passion, extreme excitement causes sodium loss. Self-abuse and self-hatred also cause loss of sodium.

You will also lose sodium when you have an acid body. Sodium is used to neutralize acids and is used up when you have an excess to neutralize.

Sodium also maintains your cell permeability. It moves into your cells, and out of your cells as it transports sugars and amino acids into your cells. It is involved in muscle contractions.

Sodium is also found in the blood, and there it functions to keep other minerals soluble, so that they do not precipitate out to form deposits. It helps to move carbon dioxide out of your body and is involved in the production of HCL acid in your stomach. It provides a protective layer in your stomach so that HCL does not create ulcers in your stomach lining.

A deficiency in sodium can also result in decreased iron chemical activity. Sodium is needed so that your body can use iron.

Daily Sodium Requirements

You only need around 500 milligrams of sodium per day, but most people who do not watch their salt use get around 4400 to 8800 milligram per day. Since sodium attracts water, eating high levels of sodium each day usually leads to high blood pressure due to extra water in the blood vessels.

Sodium Bicarbonate

Sodium bicarbonate, NaHCO3, or sodium hydrogen carbonate is the common baking soda, and many people know this better as Alka-Seltzer. You can use sodium bicarbonate for stomach indigestion for a short time. However, using it long-term to alleviate your stomach problems can result in side effects. It is also used to make your blood or urine less acidic.

When sodium bicarbonate is used long term, the bicarbonate part of this chemical, HCO3, is readily absorbed into the body causing a pH change in your body. This change in pH result in a condition called Systemic Alkalosis.

Systemic Alkalosis is a condition where excess bicarbonate ions are in your tissue causing the pH to exceed 7.4. This is the opposite of having an acid body and is a condition where there is an excess of alkaline ions throughout your body. Normally, the kidneys will excrete the excess bicarbonate, but there are a few conditions that prevent the kidney from removing the excess bicarbonate, which then leads to Systemic Alkalosis.

One of the effects of alkalosis is an excess of sodium in your body, which comes from the sodium bicarbonate and puts your body's pH out of balance. When you have an excess of sodium in your body, it can lead to a variety of various body conditions – edema, high blood pressure, or cell malfunction.

Some of the side effects of prolong use of sodium bicarbonate, which come from the bicarbonate are:

severe headache or nausea

loss of appetite
irritability or weakness
frequent urge to urinate
swelling of legs for feet
dark or bloody stools
Blood in urine

Taking sodium bicarbonate pills to relieve an acid body is not recommended.   This compound should not be used for medical purposes without direction from a doctor.

Chapter 7: Activities Of Sodium In Your Body

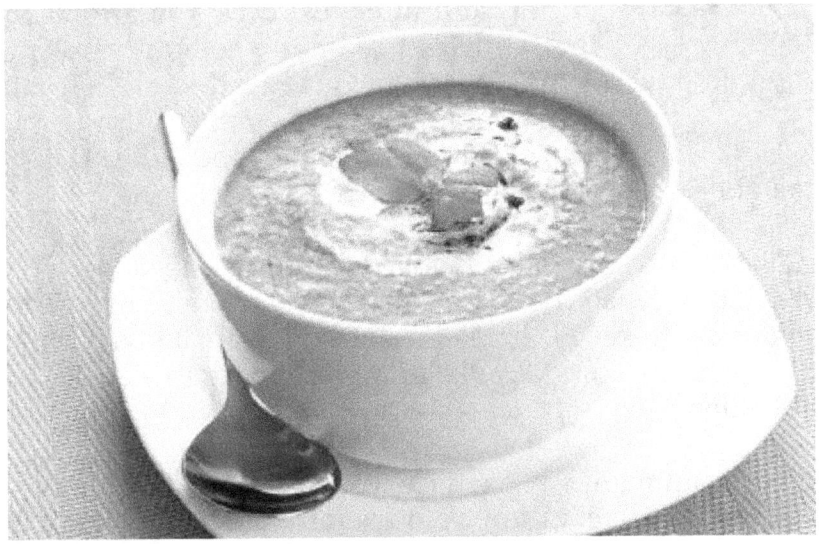

Organic Sodium helps to keep calcium in solution. When your body lacks sodium, calcium will precipitate from solution and create calcium crystals in different parts of your body. When you eat table salt, your body removes calcium from your body and excretes it in your urine.

What you eat and absorb will determine what amount of sodium your body has. The actual sodium requirement of each person differs based on age and size. You need less than 3 grams of sodium daily, but the average American diet provides around six gram. It's the kidneys that help to keep excess sodium out of your body, by excreting it in your urine. Other parts of your body will also eliminate sodium – skin, colon, and all liquid discharges.

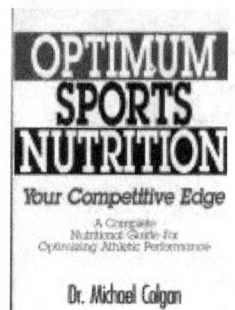

OPTIMUM SPORTS NUTRITION

Your Competitive Edge

A Complete
Nutritional Guide for
Optimizing Athletic Performance

Dr. Michael Colgan

In his book, Dr. Colgan, Michael, Optimum Sports Nutrition, New York, Advanced Research Press, 1993 say, "From all the ads for electrolyte replacement drinks for use during and after exercise, you would think that athletes need more sodium. Except for some ultra-distance athletes (Ironman length triathlons, 100-mile running races) that's just promotional flapdoodle. The human body conserves its electrolytes."

Dr Colgan says that after exercise, you don't need electrolytes or sodium because you lose water during exercise by sweating, but your body keeps the electrolytes in your body. You only need to drink water, because now your water to electrolytes is out of balance.

In the beginning of any exercise, you lose some sodium in your sweat, but as you continue your exercise or sport, your body at some point starts to conserve your sodium. The result is that you don't lose much sodium as has been previous thought by many doctors, sports people or people. You don't need those sports drinks that say brings your electrolytes back to normal, when you are working or playing hard.

Sodium and water go together. Sodium attracts water. So if your sodium intake increases, your body will retain more water. The more sodium you have in your body the more water you need to balance this sodium.

When you get thirsty, the posterior pituitary gland will release an anti-diuretic hormone, so that your kidney does not excrete too much water to your bladder. This will help you to maintain the water you have in your body.

When your body sodium decreases, your thirst disappears, the anti-diuretic hormone is suppressed, and the kidney excretes more liquid into your bladder. The result is your body starts to excrete the excess water.

In some cases, you can have an excess of sodium in your body. People who are overweight should decrease their intake of sodium, since sodium attracts water and can add body weight. Excess sodium has been also associated with a higher risk of cancer, since it upsets the sodium potassium balance. People who eat a diet of high salted foods such as fish, pork, or dried meat upset the sodium potassium balance. The sodium potassium balance is required, since it is these two elements that maintain the right electrical voltage across your body cells. When this voltage is upset, it leads to disease.

What Sodium Does In Your Body

As was mention, one of the key functions of sodium is to maintain your water balance throughout your body and in this process, it helps to keep your cells healthy. It is also involved in neutralizing acid molecules that accumulate in your body, from the food you eat, the polluted air you breathe, the negative thoughts you have, or the bad water you drink.

How Sodium Keeps Cells Functioning

Understanding one portion of how your cells work through the use of sodium and potassium is an important step in knowing why you should strive to eat the right sodium foods. This includes not eating an excess of table salt.

Sodium is found outside and inside of your cells. Fifty percent of that sodium is in your extracellular fluid, outside of your cells, 10% inside of your cells, and 40% in your bones. Typically, there are 7% sodium ions inside your cells and 93% outside your cells.

Your size and age determine how much sodium your body needs. What you eat and how you absorb your food will determine how much sodium goes into your body.

Typically, your body needs around 200mg to 500 mg of sodium daily, but it has been found that people intake up to 6000 mg daily. If you have normal functioning kidneys, the amount of sodium maintained in your body is constant. The kidneys will excrete excess sodium from your body. Sodium is also excreted in feces and sweat.

In your body, sodium and water balance each other. If you eat too much sodium, the water in your body will increase. If you eat less sodium, the amount of water held in the extracellular fluids will decrease.

Your body controls the amount of water you maintain in your body by a diuretic and anti-diuretic hormone that is released to pass more water out of your kidney as urine or not to pass water out of your body. When your sodium level increases, your body makes you thirsty so you will drink more water.

Sodium Potassium Pump

Sodium and potassium ions exist outside your cells, extracellular liquid, and inside your cells, intracellular liquid. In the cell, there is around 7% sodium and 92% potassium. Outside the cell, they are the opposite, 93% sodium and 8% potassium. These are the percentages that should be maintained for good cellular function. Naturally, sodium tends to diffuse into the cell while potassium tends to diffuse out of the cell.

The sodium-potassium pump is embedded in the cell membrane and opens to move sodium or potassium ions back and forth across from outside to inside or from inside to outside the cells. This is done to keep a certain voltage across the cell membrane. This potential allows sugar or glucose and amino acids to move into the cell using the sodium-potassium pump. As cells use up the nutrients, you eat, toxic by products are created. These products are then transported out of the cell using the sodium-potassium pump.

Go to the following link to view sodium pump process.

http://url2it.com/msrc

or

http://url2it.com/msrd
So now you can see the importance of maintain the proper levels of sodium in your body.

Chapter 8: Detrimental Effects of Table Salt To Avoid

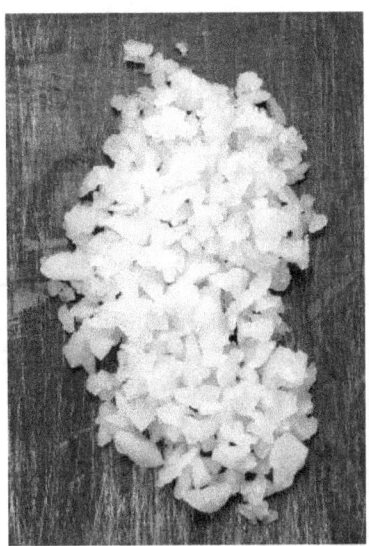

Your body does not need table salt. But it does need sodium and chloride, which is found naturally in food. Your body stores sodium and has plenty, if you eat the right kind of food. When you have a poor diet or have a destructive lifestyle, you deplete your sodium.

There are many detrimental effects of eating too much table salt. However, these effects are not related to the sodium you get from the food you eat. This is because the sodium you get from natural food, which has not been cooked, is electrically charged and has energy associated with it. Table salt is a dead food and has no electrical charge associated with it.

Bone Density

When you eat salt, calcium is excreted from your body and this leads to lower bone density. Granted, the amount of calcium loss is small, but over time, it can be significant. If you drink coffee, then caffeine will cause you to lose a bit more bone density.

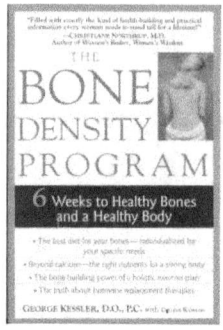

In his book, Kessler, George D.O., P.C. and Kapklein, Colleen, The Bone Density Program, New York, Ballantine Books, 2000, he points out that, "As with high blood pressure, some people seem to be more sensitive to the effects of salt that others. But, the group of sensitive people is large enough that everyone would be wise to use discretion when it comes to salt. Since you don't automatically know whether you are sensitive... Stay within the American Heart Association's guidelines (2,000 mg a day or less) to be safe."

Heart Disease and Cancer

Many studies have been done on how salt contributes to heart disease and cancer. It has been thought that high salt diets contribute to heart diseases.

But, in Dr. Watts, L. David, Trace Elements and Other Essential Nutrients, Texas, 4th Writer's B-L-O-C-K, 2003, he clarifies studies that point to chlorine as the major contributor to heart and cancer diseases.

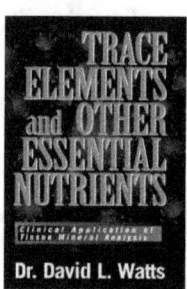

"It now appears that the salt-hypertension link was overly exaggerated. In fact, stringent salt restriction is only necessary for a small segment of the affected population. Only about 10-15 percent may benefit from limiting salt intake. These are a group of individuals with high blood pressure who are classified as 'salt-sensitive.' More recent studies implicate chloride in the development of hypertension rather than sodium alone. Animal studies have shown that high amounts of sodium chloride can induce an elevation in blood pressure."

The actual cause of high blood pressure is not that clear cut, since many people with high blood pressure may have a number of mineral imbalances. Some people are sensitive to sodium and some to chloride and these sensitivities can cause various health issues.

Another factor involved in heart disease is the sodium to potassium ratio. Dr. Julian Whitaker, M.D. points out that most people have a ratio of twice as much sodium as potassium in the body. By changing this ratio, Dr. Whitaker claims you can protect yourself from heart and cancer. To do this you need to watch your salt intake and learn which foods give you more potassium and add them to your diet.

Excess salt has also been known as a stomach cancer threat. This is especially true when the sodium in salt combines with other carcinogens – barbecue smoke, grilled meat, sodium nitrides, or pesticides. Salt irritates the stomach, which increases the disposition of precancerous cell replication and powers chemical carcinogen to do more stomach damage. When your diet is low in fruits and vegetables, the results of a high salt diet are even more damaging.

Kidney Damage

When you eat salt, your body tries to get rid of it. It does this by making you thirsty. If you drink more water, your kidney will cause you to urinate more. This is how your body tries to get rid of the salt you eat.

Of all your body organs, your kidneys suffer the most when you eat salt. If you eat more salt than your kidneys can remove, your kidneys break down the salt and deposit it in various parts of your body, but mostly in your lower legs. Then, your body tries to protect itself from this salt by bringing water to that area. This causes swelling in the legs and feet. This also causes puffy eyelids and bags underneath your eyes.

Fluid Retention and Sodium Restricted diet

In cases where excess sodium has been consumed and where the kidney has not expelled the excess, fluid retention disease starts to appear, if the excess sodium condition continues to exist. Fluid retention diseases are congestive heart failure and edema. Other excess sodium conditions are kidney failure, adrenal disease, and cirrhosis of the liver. Under these conditions, a sodium restricted diet is called for. Using the information in this kindle e-book provides you with a good start in restricting your use of table salt in your diet.

Chapter 9: Sodium Diet Foods You Must Eat

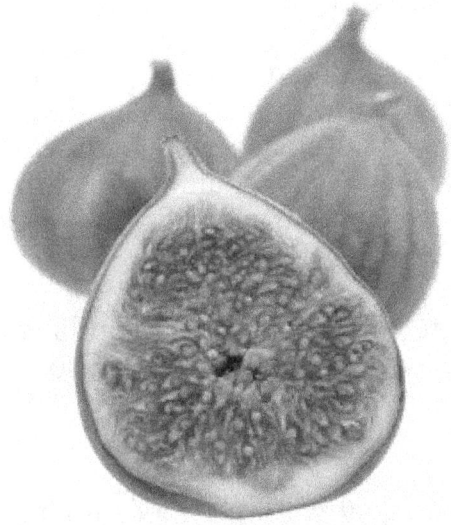

When joints start to get hard and painful to move, they lack nutrients or specific minerals. With arthritis, sodium is lacking, so sodium foods recommended are okra and celery, which are also available in tablets. Goat whey is another good source of sodium and can be purchased on the internet. To get more information on goat whey, just type this word into Google search.

Other fruits and vegetables that are high in sodium should also be eaten. Only fruits that are picked ripe should be eaten. If they are picked green and allowed to become ripe, they will not have as much sodium, since the sun helps to create the sodium in food.

Some people who have symptoms related to sodium deficiencies may recover quickly or may take a long time to benefit from the addition of sodium. It takes up to 3 months to replenish the sodium reserves in your body, when they are low. And this is providing you are eating an excess of fruits and vegetables.

Sodium and the stomach

The stomach is considered a sodium organ, since it stores sodium in its walls to prevent stomach acid from burning a hole in its tissue. As stomach HCl, hydrochloric acid, moves against your stomach walls, sodium neutralizes it, preventing it from damaging your stomach walls.

The sodium you eat first goes through the stomach walls and the excess goes to the joints. So, if you have joint problems, you most likely have stomach problems also.

Sodium Foods

Raw goat milk and goat whey are foods high in sodium. Black mission figs are also high in sodium.

Here is a broth that you can make to get extra sodium and potassium called Veal Joint Broth as described by Bernard Jensen, Ph.D.

"Use a clean, fresh, uncut veal joint and after washing in cold water, put into a large cooking pot: cover half with water and add the following vegetables and greens cut up finely:

Small stalk of celery
1 ½ cups apple peelings, ½ in thick
2 cups potato peeing, ½ in thick
½ cup chopped parsley
2 beets, grated
1 large parsnip
1 onion

½ cup okra

Simmer all ingredients for 4 or 5 hours: strain off liquid and discard solid ingredients. There should be 1 ½ quarts of liquid. Drink hot or cold and keep refrigerated."

These are the foods high in sodium:

Apples	kale	kelp	lentils
Dried apricots	asparagus	barley	raw milk
Beets	mustard greens	greens	beets
Red cabbage	okra	carrots	parsley
Celery	dried pea's	cheeses	chickpeas
Red peppers	coconut	prunes	raisins
Collard	sesame	spinach	dates
Dulse	strawberries	egg yolks	sunflower
Figs	Swiss chard	turnips	goat milk
Artichokes	lemons	parsley	watercress

Every day you should be eating these various vegetables. You want to make sure you eat at least three highly colored vegetables with your lunch and dinner – bright green, red, orange, yellow, purple and so on. The more colors you can include in your meals the healthier you will be.

Minimize Your Use Of Salt

Since you have probably been using salt for a long time, you have become accustom to having a lot of salt in your food. You can use other ways to spice up your food, without using a lot of salt. Here are a few ways to do this.

Use herbs, spices, and culinary herbs

Use lemon or lime juice to flavor your food

Don't use salt in cooking nor have it on your table

Use butter that is salt free. Don't use margarine, since it has trans fatty acids or hydrogenated oils.

Most canned foods or processed foods are high in sodium. Look for those are low sodium or sodium free.

Choose breakfast cereals that are low in sodium

Fresh meat, poultry, fish are low in sodium, avoid the processed meats

Use low sodium soy sauce

Avoid teriyaki sauce and miso sauce, which are very high in sodium

Avoid boiling vegetable with salt added, vegetables will absorb the salt

Use these labels to determine how much sodium is in food you buy per serving.

Sodium – Free, contains less than five mg of sodium.
Very low sodium contains less than 34 mg of sodium.
Low – sodium has less than 141 mg of sodium.
Reduced – sodium has 75% of sodium found in normal food.

Salt Replacement

You can eliminate the need to use salt in your food preparation or reduce its use to a very low amount. This is done by becoming familiar with spices and culinary herbs. By consistently using herbs and spices you get fantastic good taste and their therapeutically benefits. The best way to use herbs and spices is to read about their use in food and create a blend that you can use over and over.

Here are some spices to consider:

Basil – use in tomato sauces, soups, salads. Place a small amount in your palm then rub both hands to break the tiny flakes and let them fall into your soup.

Cloves – use with pumpkin and squash dishes or to spice up your rice and baked goods dishes.

Garlic – is part of the onion family, and it should be used every day and in as many different dishes that you prepare.

Ginger – use it in cooking meat, stir fry, cookies, or cakes.

Paprika – use it to liven up chicken, mashed potatoes or broiled fish.

Red pepper powder – use it in soups, stews, sauces. You can use a variety of different pepper powders. Try the Eagle brand chili powder, which contains more than one type of chili pepper.

Rosemary – used to flavor chicken, turkey, and lamb.

Turmeric – use with curries.

You can get fresh herbs such as basil, dill, parsley, cilantro or mint. Put the dried herbs into your pot early in your cooking. For fresh herbs, wait until near the end of your cooking.

One of the ways to use herbs is to create a blend that you can add to your dishes as you cook them. You can create a blend for different types of dishes that you cook. Through experimenting with different herbs and spice you can make your own blends. Here are a couple of simple blends.

For Italian Dishes – use only the amount you need.

1 tablespoon of dried oregano
1 tablespoon dried basil
1 tablespoon of dried thyme

For **Mexican soups** add these herbs together.

1 tablespoon of dried oregano
1 tablespoon of basil
1 tablespoon of chili powder
1 tablespoon of a variety of chili powders
1/2 tablespoon of cumin

A **general blend** would be like this.

1 tablespoon of dried basil
2 teaspoons of celery seed
2 teaspoons of dried savory
1 teaspoon of dried thyme
1 teaspoon of dried marjoram

Sodium bicarbonate

Organic Sodium bicarbonate, $NaHCO_3$, contains sodium, hydrogen, carbon and oxygen and is also known as baking soda. Organic sodium bicarbonate is created in your body and is used when you have mucus congestions in the throat and bronchial areas. When you have these conditions, sodium foods are recommended. Bicarbonate is also called for to reduce gout, diabetic acid, sub acid blood, and stomach mucus.

Saliva

Saliva is an alkaline substance, which is used to neutralize acids as they enter your mouth. It is composed of many different alkaline compounds, such as calcium, sodium, and magnesium phosphates, sodium and potassium chlorides, and sodium carbonate.

Sodium is involved in a variety of digestion processes as food goes into your mouth, stomach and small intestine.

Bile

Your bile that comes from your liver into your gallbladder consists of:

Sodium carbonate
Sodium phosphate
Potassium chloride
Sodium chloride
Lecithin
Sodium palmitate
Sodium stearate
Cholesterin
Sodium taurocholate
Sodium glycocholate
Water

When your body doesn't have enough sodium, it will take it from your bile in the gallbladder and as sodium is depleted from the bile, cholesterol will precipitate causing gallstones.
Bile is necessary for you to have regular bowel movements, since it stimulates peristaltic colon action. When your liver is not putting out enough bile, you will have constipation. When you have enough bile your stool will be a light brown.

Hidden Salt

There are many processed foods that contain sodium chloride or inorganic salt. This is the type of salt that creates sickness, when consumed in excess. As you look at the various foods you buy, look at the nutritional label and buy only those foods that have less salt.

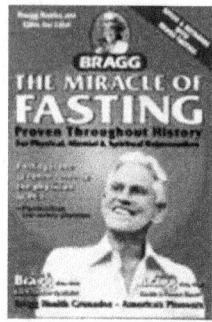 In his Bragg Health Series, N.D., PhD, Bragg, G., Paul and Bragg Patricia, N.D., PhD, The Miracle of Fasting, California, Health Science, they recall an incident that shows the deadly power of salt, "The most dramatic wrongful death case against salt occurred in a Binghamton, New York hospital, where a number of babies died when salt was inadvertently used in their formula.

An overdose of salt can kill a baby quickly. The body needs natural, organic sodium – not table salt, an inorganic chemical. You can obtain natural sodium which Mother Nature provides in organic form in celery, beets, carrots, potatoes, soybeans, turnips sea vegetation, seaweed, kelp, watercress, etc. and many other natural healthy foods. Remember, only organic minerals can be utilized by your body's living cells."

The amount of organic sodium you need per day is up to 500mg. But because there is hidden salt in most processed foods and by your use of table salt, you probable consume from 500 to 6000 mg per day.

Here are a few of the foods with hidden salt to look out for:

Cured meats – bacon, hot dogs, sliced processed meats, sausages

Canned soups, canned tuna, prepared pancakes
TV dinners
Regular soy sauce
Tomato sauces
All packaged foods

Sodium in your drinking water

There is also sodium in the bottled water that you drink. The amount it has is based on the brand. Some bottled water has very little and others have up to 200 mg or more. If you are on a strict sodium diet, then you need to know which bottled water has less sodium.

Most bottle water companies put sodium into their water so that it tastes better. But, some do not and just allow what is in the water to exist. Companies that produce low –salt or no-salt water must list the sodium contain in their bottles.

Water that is labeled Natural Spring Water has sodium, but this type of water has the lowest sodium content as compared to other bottled water. If you drink distilled water then there is no sodium in this type of water.

Sodium Compounds Which Attack Your Immune System

Sodium can form many compound inside and outside your body. Many food suppliers tend to put a variety of sodium compounds in your food to make it taste better or to have a better consistency. These compounds tend to erode cells and tissue creating clumps of deadly free radicals. The result of this is that they use up a lot of your antioxidants that you need elsewhere in your body.

Here is a list of these sodium compounds that you want to

avoid. Read the labels on the food you buy and check that the food you buy is free of these compounds.

Salt, sodium chloride – is a destructive compound, which you should eat less of. Get your sodium by eating more sodium foods.

Baking powder – used in various baking products.

Baking soda, sodium bicarbonate – used to relieve various stomach issues.

Brine, table salt or water – used in foods to control growth of bacteria and in cleaning fruits and vegetables, in freezing or canning certain foods, and for flavoring corned beef, pickles, sauerkraut, French fries.

Disodium phosphate – used in quick-cooking cereals or processed cheeses

Monosodium glutamate - comes in many different brands, used in packaged or frozen foods.

Sodium alginate – used in some chocolate milks and ice cream
Sodium benzoate – used as a preservative in sauces and salad dressings

Sodium hydroxide – used to soften olives, hominy and some fruits and vegetables.

Sodium propionate – used in pasteurized cheeses, some breads and cakes to inhibit mold.

Sodium sulfite – used to bleach fruits for artificial colors, such as cherries, dried fruit.

Sodium nitrate or sodium nitrite – a dangerous preservative that is used on meat, which is considered carcinogen, cancer forming.

Sodium citrate – a chemical used in food that is harmful to your health.

Sodium dioctyl sulfate, Colace, – used as a lubricant in laxative products and can be habit forming.

Chapter 10: Salt Bath Curative Effects

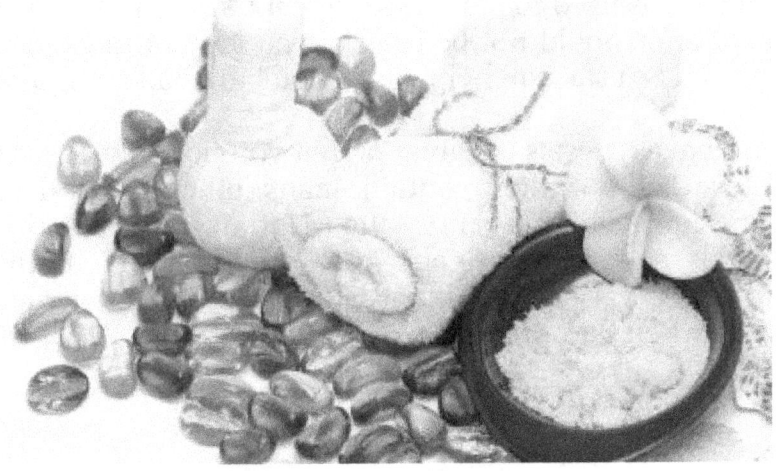

External Use Of Salt

Eating sodium is not the only way to get it into your body. It can be used externally as a natural remedy. Salt can be used in many ways to heal and detoxify your body. In combination with water, salt can be applied externally and have a positive effect on your body's pH and health. It is recommended that you use coarse salt or sea salt for your footbath, tub bath, or massage.

The types of salts below can be found by searching on Google. Type in coarse salt and get a variety of sites that sell this type of salt and many others that you can use for your bath.

Here some of the different types of salts you can use:

Himalayan Crystal Salt, food grade
Coarse sea salt
Dead Sea Bath Salt -
Epson Salt
Atlantic Sea Bath Salt

Epson salt is used to create strong perspiration. It is a muscle relaxer and should not be used, if you are not in good health. The Dead Sea salt can help you, if you have had an injury.

What makes these salts great is that you not only have regular salt, $NaCl_2$, but they contain many other mineral salts – magnesium and potassium salts. Not all salts have the same minerals, so you have to check the specifications. Using salts that have a variety of minerals is a great way to get curative effects, when they are used as massage or bath.

Salt Massage Bath

You will want to do a salt massage bath, when you want to stop an oncoming cold, relieve gout pain, restore blood and lymph circulation, overcome sluggishness, and to clean your skin of dirt and dead skin.

This type of massage will improve your mood and reduce your stress as the friction of the salt goes over your skin. It acts as a skin and body stimulant, by increasing blood circulation. If you have a mild case of depression this will help you.

Here's how to do it. Use plain coarse salt, sea salt, or many of the other salts.

Create a slushy salt paste with warm water. You can sit in the tub or shower and pour some salt and water into your hands and create a paste. Apply this paste all over your body from shoulders to feet in a slow circular motion. If you want you can place your feet in hot water as you massage your body. Do the massage only for a few minutes.

After your massage, wash off salt with a gentle shower of slightly warm water and rub your skin with a sponge to remove the salt and stimulate your skin.

If you have any open cuts do not do the salt massage in those areas. Also, if you have skin lesions or skin inflammation, do not do the massage.

Complete immersion Salt Bath

Use a salt bath when you need to relax. If you have been sitting in your chair all day and have had anxiety, then a salt bath will help you release tension. If you need to clean your skin of dirt or dead skin, a salt bath will help you do this. Women in menopause will benefit for a salt bath.

Here how to do it.

In a tub of warm water put 1 to 2 cups of salt crystals. The more cups you use, the more you will perspire. To simulate sea water, you can use 5 pounds of coarse salt, and this will act as a mild tonic on your body.

You can use water at 65 to 75 F for your bath but stay in the bath for 2 minutes or so. With warmer water, you can stay in the bath for up to 15 minutes. Finish your bath with a warm shower and rub your body with a sponge or cloth.

Chapter 11: Sodium Gives You An Alkaline Body

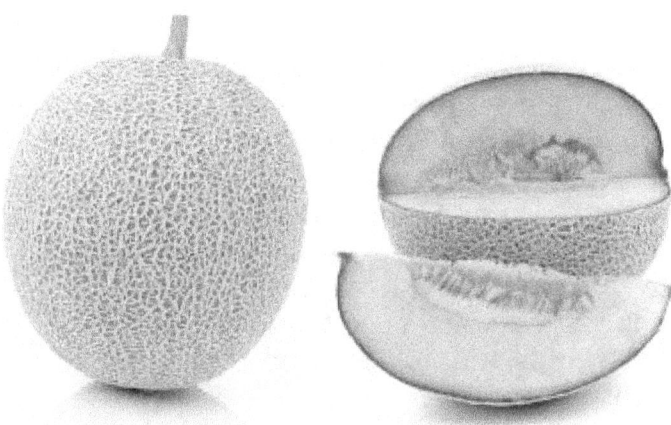

A diet rich in sodium provides the body with the sodium to neutralize acids in your kidney and liver. Sodium works to eliminate acetic, buturic, lactic and other fatty acids, which are derived from starchy foods, lard, margarine, potatoes, oily nuts, and meats. These foods cause the precipitation of sodium and potassium and deplete them, if you continually eaten them.

When sodium is deficient, bad bacteria takes over your digestive tract. In the colon, sodium keeps the environment slightly alkaline to control the bad bacterial.

Sodium Deficiencies

Here are some of the symptoms you will have if you have a deficiency of body sodium:

Gout	cracking joints	excess mucus
Dull complexion	tendons stiff	bloating
Restless nerves	fatigue	constipation
Mental confusion	drowsiness	Frontal headache
Bad breath	Lack of saliva	white coated tongue

Because fruits and vegetables are naturally grown from soil, they pull minerals out of the ground and can be a great source of minerals like sodium for you. Because of these minerals and other nutrients, fruits and vegetables have amazing curative effects, when they are eaten raw.

If you have an acid body, like most people do, this is what is causing your illness. You need to move your acid body into an alkaline condition and sodium and other minerals can help you to do this.

Minerals

Moving your body more toward alkalinity is what will give you the best curative effects of fruits. An alkaline body prevents your body from becoming ill and forming deadly diseases, like all kinds of joint problems, organ degradation, body pain, or even cancer. If you are already sick, then all the chemicals inside fruits will help to revive you to better health. This is provided that your tissue damage has not gone beyond repair.

The minerals most important in changing and maintaining your body in an alkaline condition are sodium, potassium, chloride, calcium, phosphorus, magnesium, and sulfur.

Now, how your body can become alkaline might become a little confusing at first because of the terms used, but let's break this down into small parts. This process has been discussed in previous chapters, but this explanation gives more details. First, we are going to be defining some terms, so we can then start talking the same language.

Acid Binding

There are certain minerals that are called acid binding. And these are minerals, as mentioned earlier, are the most important ones in fruits, Sodium, potassium, chloride, calcium, phosphorus, magnesium, because they are acid binding.

What acid binding means is when you eat fruits with these minerals, your cells, after metabolism, create an alkaline ash. This ash will seek out acids in your body and bind with them to neutralize them.

Alkaline Ash

Now, that this alkaline forming ash has tied up an acid it is carried to the kidney where it is expelled as urine.

Different reactions can occur when an acid binding mineral, like say sodium, encounters an acid. Of course, acids in the body are toxic, so the body has the priority of getting rid of them fast, since they can damage tissue and cause pain and disease.

Here is another path way of the acid binding mineral process when it combines with an acid.

The Acid Binding Mineral Process

When you eat acid binding food, the blood carries it to the cells where it is oxidized, digested, or metabolized. The result of this digestion is a carbonic acid salt of alkaline minerals, which reacts with body acids and binds with them. In this process, a weak carbonic acid is created. Now, this weak carbonic acid is taken by the blood into the lungs where it is released as carbon dioxide and water.

If not all the acid toxins are captured by acid binding matter, the remaining acids can be neutralized by body stores of alkaline minerals. If you don't have a good store of alkaline minerals, then these acids will remain in your body creating pain and disease.

But, if you do have a good store of alkaline minerals, then these minerals will find these acids, capture them and bind with them. Then these acids are routed out through your urine or colon and out of your body.

So you can see the importance of getting a lot of alkaline minerals into your body. Without them, acids which do not get bonded to alkaline minerals would move back into body tissue and continue their body damage.

Alkaline Binding

Now, there are also minerals that become alkaline binding and these minerals are sulphur, chlorine, iodine, phosphorous, bromine, fluorine, copper, and silicon.

It is these minerals that when digested by a cell will produce an acid salt that will bind with alkaline minerals. These minerals will be excreted through your urine. When alkaline minerals are bonded to an acid salt, the alkaline mineral is removed from your body, and your body becomes more acidic, the condition you are trying to avoid.

Although you need to eat both foods that are acid binding or alkaline binding, you want to eat more of the acid binding food.

Final Comments – The Secrets of Sodium

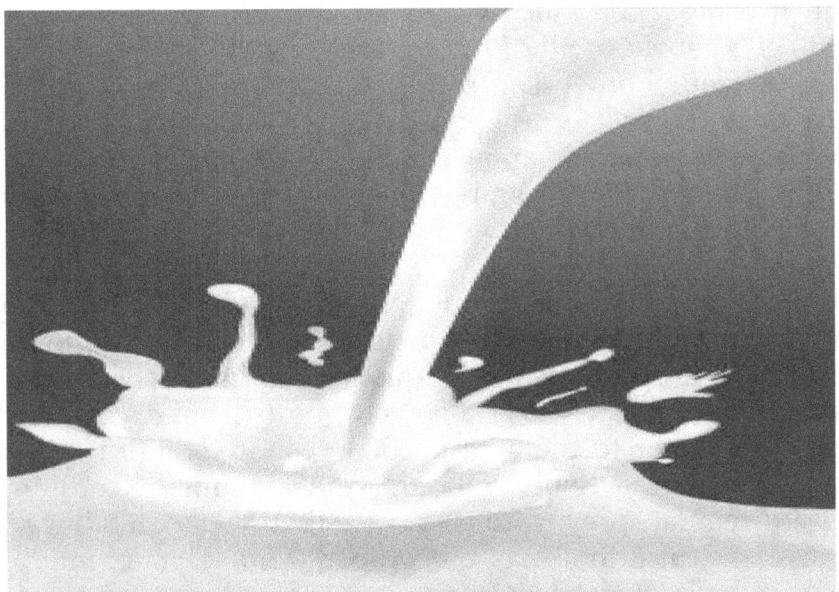

The difference between organic sodium and inorganic sodium is critical to understand and apply. Organic sodium is only found in natural produce and is available to you when you eat fresh produce. When this produce is stored and sprayed for storage and transport, it loses is potential to provide you with the best sodium and other minerals.

Your body only uses organic sodium because it has electrical energy in the form of ions and frequency. The frequency come from its color, and it is this energy that the cells use to provide you with the energy you need to run your body.

Whereas inorganic sodium is in table salt, and this is the type of sodium that you find in most grocery store package products. When you eat table salt your body tries to get rid of it. This is why sodium attracts so much water. Through water, your body can eliminate this salt in your urine.

But, if you eat too much salt, your kidneys are overwhelmed and can't get rid of all of it. So, it stores this salt in different parts of your body. The result is that you gain weight and develop sickness. Excess body water creates edema. In your cells, excess water will appear, and now the electrical potential that is between outside and the inside your cell is changed and your cell will not work properly.

Organic sodium is used throughout your body, and it first goes to your stomach walls where it is stored to prevent the high stomach acid from burning a hole in your stomach - stomach ulcers. Then it is used to keep your joints from drying out by attracting water to the area needed. Since sodium is part of the Potassium – Sodium Pump, the amount of sodium is closely regulated by your body so that you don't have an excess. Natural food has the proper ratio of potassium and sodium the body needs.

An excess of sodium attracts water, and excess water will cause your body cells to function less efficiently. When you are deficient in sodium, you will have a variety of symptoms and illnesses that will start to develop. You can maintain adequate supply of sodium in your body, by eating raw fruits and vegetables and goat whey.

Most likely, you will not have an excess of salt, unless you eat a lot of salty meats and use plenty of salt with your meals. Since your body uses sodium to reduce acids in your body, sodium is used up quickly and your sodium reserves can become depleted.

Most people have acid bodies and that's one reason they have various illnesses. What this means is that they are deficient in organic sodium and they are not able to neutralize all the acid that is created in their body from the acid foods that they eat. Acid foods like meat, potatoes, butter, carbohydrates need to be balanced with alkaline foods, like fruits and vegetables.

To understand how to change an acid body to an alkaline body check my kindle book called, "ALKALINE BODY - HOW TO CHANGE AN ACID BODY INTO AN ALKALINE BODY"

Here is something for you to do to get more natural sodium into your body. Go to the Internet and look up goat milk and goat whey. Read about the benefits you can get by using these products. Then the next time you go to a health-food store see if they have raw goat milk or goat whey.

They might have raw goat milk depending on what state you live in and mostly likely you can only find goat whey on the internet as "whex." Goat milk is an alkaline food and has a lot of sodium. Even raw cow's milk is alkaline, but when it is pasteurized or homogenized it becomes an acid food.

Appendix A: Choosing The Best Sodium Foods

Here is a more comprehensive list of foods and the amount of sodium they contain. This is based on 3 1/2 cups of the food. This list is to give you an idea of the amount of sodium in both processed foods and fruits and vegetables. You should pick those foods that are more natural and that are not processed, which have the highest sodium value. Those foods with high potassium value are also important.

Meat and Poultry*	Portion	Sodium (mg.)	Potassium (mg.)
Bacon	1 strip (1 oz.	71	16
Beef			
Corned Beef(canned)	3 slices	803	51
Hamburger	¼ lb.	41	382
Pot Roast (rump)	¼ lb.	43	309
Sirloin Steak	½ lb.	57	545
Chicken (broiler)	3\12 oz.	78	320
Duck	3\12 oz.	82	285
Frankfurter (all beef)	1/8 lb.	550	110
Ham	1/4 lb.	37	260
Fresh			
Cured, butt	1/4 lb.	518	239
Cured, shank	1/4 lb.	336	155
Lamb			
Shoulder Chop (1)	½ lb.	72	422
Rib Chop (2)	½ lb.	68	398
Leg Roast	¼ lb.	68	398
Liver		41	246
Beef	31/2 oz.	86	325
Calf	31/2 oz.	131	436
Pork			
Loin Chop	6 oz.	52	500

Spareribs (3 or 4)	31/2 oz.	51	360
Sausage (link or bulk)	31/2 oz.	740	140
Turkey	31/2oz.		
Veal		40	320
Cutlet	6 oz.	6	448
Loin Chop (1)	1/2 lb.	4	384
Rump Roast	¼ lb.	6	244
Fish			
Clams (4 1g.,9 sm.)	31/2 oz.	36	235
Cod	31/2 oz.	70	382
Flounder or Sole	31/2 oz.	56	366
Lobster (1)			
Boiled, with			
2 tbsp. butter	3/4lb.	210	180
Oysters (5 to 8)			
Fresh	31/2 oz.	73	121
Frozen	31/2 oz.	380	210
Salmon (pink, canned)	31/2 oz.	387	361
Sardines (8) Canned, in oil)	31/2 oz.	510	560
Shrimp	31/2oz.	140	220
Tuna			
Canned, in oil	31/2 oz.	800	301
Canned, in water	31/2oz.	41	279
Snacks			
Candy			
Chocolate Creams	1 candy	1	15
Milk Chocolate	1 oz.	30	105
Ice Cream			
Chocolate	½ pint	75	*
Vanilla	½ pint	82	210
Nuts			
Cashews (roasted)			
Peanuts (roasted)	6-8	2	84
Salted	1 tbsp.	69	105
Unsalted	1 tbsp.	Trace	111
Olives			
Green	2 medium	312	7
Ripe	2 large	150	5
Potato Chips	5 chips	34	88

Pretzels (3 ring)	1 average	87	7
Dairy Products			
Butter (salted)	1 pat	99	2
Butter (unsalted)	1 pat	1	2
Cheese			
American, cheddar	1 oz.	197	23
American processed	1 oz.	318	22
Cottage, creamed	31/2 oz.	299	85
Cream (heavy)	1 tbsp.	35	10
Egg	1 large	66	70
Milk (whole)	8 oz.	122	352
Oleomargarine (salted)	1 pat	99	1
Breads Cereals, Etc.			
Bread			
Rye 1 slice	128	33	56
White (enriched)	slice	177	20
Whole Wheat	1 slice	121	63
Corn Flakes	cup	165	40
Macaroni (enriched, cooked tender)	1 cup	1	85
Noodles (enriched, cooked)	1 cup	3	70
Oatmeal (cooked)	1 cup	1	130
Rice (white, dry)	¼ cup	3	45
Spaghetti (enriched, cooked tender)	1 cup	2	92
Waffles (enriched)	1 waffle	356	109
Wheat Germ	3 tbsp. 1	232	102
Beverages			
Apple Juice	6 oz.	2	187
Beer	8 oz.	8	46
Coca-Cola	6 oz.	2	88
Coffee (brewed)	1 cup	3	149
Cranberry Cocktail	7 oz.	2	20
Ginger Ale	8 oz.	18	1
Orange Juice			
Canned	8 oz.	3	500
Fresh	8 oz.	3	496
Prune Juice	6 oz.	4	423
Tea	8 oz.	2	21
Fruits*			

Apple	1 medium	1	165
Apricot Fresh	2-3	1	281
Canned (in syrup)	3 halves	1	234
Dried	17 halves	26	979
Fruits*			
Banana	1 6-in.	1	370
Blueberries	1 cup	1	81
Cantaloupe	¼ melon	12	251
Cherries			
Fresh	½ cup	2	191
Canned (in syrup)	½ cup	1	124
Dates			
Fresh	10 medium	1	648
Dried (pitted)	1 cup (6 oz.	2	1150
Fruit Cocktail	½ cup	5	161
Grapefruit	½ medium	1	135
Grapes	22 grapes	3	158
Orange	1 small	1	200
Peaches			
Fresh	1 medium	1	202
Canned 2 halves	2 tbsp. syru	2	130
Pears			
Fresh	½ pear	2	130
Canned 2 halves	2 tbsp. syru	1	84
Pineapple			
Fresh	¾ cup	1	146
Canned	1 slice/syru	1	96
Plums			
Fresh	2 medium	2	299
Canned	3 medium2 tbsp. syrup	1	142
Prunes			
Dried	10 large	8	694
Strawberries	10 large	1	164
Watermelon	½ cup	1	100
Vegetables*			
Artichoke			
Base and soft end of leaves	1 large bud	30	301
Asparagus			
Fresh	2/3 cup	1	183
Canned	6 spears	271	191

Beans, baked	5/8 cup	2	704
Beans, green			
Fresh	1 cup	5	189
Canned	1 cup	295	109
Beans, lima			
Fresh	5/8 cup	1	422
Canned	½ cup	271	255
Frozen	5/8 cup	129	394
Beets			
Fresh	½ cup	36	172
Canned	½ cup	196	138
Broccoli			
Fresh	2/3 cup	10	167
Brussels Sprouts	6-7 medium	10	273
Cabbage			
Raw, shredded	1 cup	20	233
Cooked	3/5 cup	14	163
Carrots			
Raw	1 large	47	341
Cooked	2/3 cup	33	222
Canned	2/3 cup	236	120
Cauliflower	7/8 cup	9	206
Celery	1 outer,3 inner stalks	63	170
Corn			
Fresh	1 medium	ear trace	196
Canned	½ cup	196	81
Cucumber, pared	½ medium	3	80
Lettuce, iceberg	3 ½ oz.	9	264
Mushrooms (uncooked)	10 sm., 41g	15	414
Vegetables*			
Onions (uncooked)	1 medium	10	157
Peas			
Fresh	2/3 cup	1	196
Canned	3/4 cup	236	96
Frozen	31/2oz.	115	135
Potatoes			
Boiled (in skin)	1 medium	3	407
French Fried	10 pieces	3	427
Radishes	10 small	18	322
Sauerkraut	2/3 cup	747	140
Spinach	½ cup	45	291

Tomatoes			
Raw	1 medium	4	366
Canned	1/2cup	130	217
Paste	31/2 oz.	38	888

About The Author And Resources

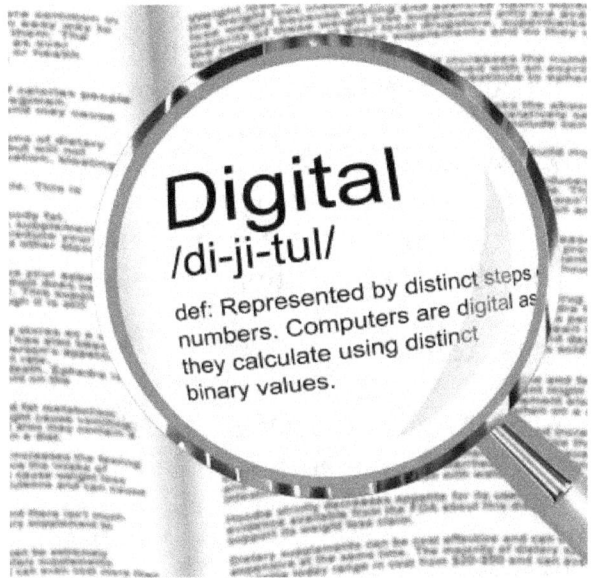

Get one of my best kindle books *free* below:

http://www.natural-remedies-thatwork.com

Rudy Silva is a natural nutritional consultant educated in the United States in Nutrition and Physics. He is a graduate from San Jose State University in California. He is author of 45 other books on natural remedies. He has authored a newsletter in natural remedies for over 10 years.

Resource page

Here are some of the other kindle e-books about natural remedies that have been written by this author. You can see the entire list at:

http://tinyurl.com/b2f7wd3

Acne Remedies
- Best natural acne treatments: Acne facial
- Effective Acne Treatments That Work

Constipation Remedies
- The Best Constipation Remedies
- Best Constipated Women Natural Cures
- How To Relieve Constipation With Fruits

Essential Fatty Acids

- Taking The Mystery Out Of Essential Fatty acids
- Amazing Fish Oil Benefits Revealed
- Omega 3 and 6 Mystery Exposed

Nutrition Remedies
- Updated Version - Secret Diet And Nutrition
- Secret Healthy Fruit Practices Revealed
- Fast Healing Juice Nutrition Therapy: Nutrition Tips 3
- Fantastic Alkaline Fruit Benefits Revealed
- Calcium (Discover How To Use Calcium To Avoid Devastating Diseases)
- Magnesium Nutrition Revealed
- Best Nutrition Health Practices
- Potassium Health Secrets Revealed
- Phosphorus, The Best Brain Food
- A Sodium Diet (What You Must Know About Sodium)
- Vegetables and Vegetable Juice Cures
- Alkaline Body: How to Change an Acid Body into an Alkaline body

Stomach Remedies
- Acid Reflux: Fast and Easy Cures For Acid Reflux
- Asthma Treatment Cures With Remedies
- How To Do Natural Colon Cleansing
- Gastrointestinal Digestion Secrets Revealed

Misc Remedies
- Natural Hair Loss Treatment: Women And Men
- Effective Natural Hemorrhoids Treatment
- Iron Deficiency Anemia
- Secrets To Understanding Behavior
- Fast Acting Ear Infection Remedies
- Best Behavior Secrets Revealed That Can Change Your Personality
- What Is A Hiatus Hernia
- Best Varicose Vein Treatments?
- Make Shampoos At Home Using Natural Ingredients:Discover recipes for quality natural hair shampoos
- How To Fix Your Thyroid Problems: Discover Hidden Ideas That Fix Your Thyroid

Minerals
- Calcium and Magnesium Magic Body Benefits Revealed
- The Magic of Sodium, Calcium and Magnesium
- Create an Alkaline Body with Potassium and Sodium: Eliminate a Potassium Deficiency
- Calcium and Phosphorus Foods: Deficiency or Excesses in These Minerals Cause Bone and Brain Power Loss
- Chlorine The Body Detoxifier (With water, chlorine will clean your body of toxins and pathogens)

Men's Health
- Best Impotence Health Diet

Weight loss
- Ten (10) Day Quick Success Weight Loss Program: A new approach to losing weight by changing your eating habits for life
- Discover Secret Anti-Aging Juice & Tonic Recipes: Unique Juices And Tonics That Create Beauty And Youth

To see all the kindle books written by this author, go to this the Authors Profile Page or this URL: http://tinyurl.com/b2f7wd3

If you need support or want to promote any of his e-books, please contact him at rss41@yahoo.com and expect a reply within 24 hours. He looks forward to hearing from you and is happy to help you understand his material on natural and nutritional health.

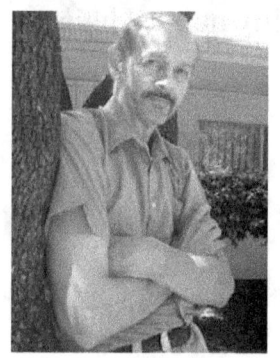

Give A Review

And, don't for get to give a review for this e-book at Amazon so that others can gain the benefits of what is in this e-book. To you, for losing weight, creating better health and more happiness in your life,

Rudy S Silva